AVOID PREPARE DEFEND

25 ESSENTIAL TIPS ON HOW TO STAY SAFE FROM CRIME

ULRICH FAIRCLOTH

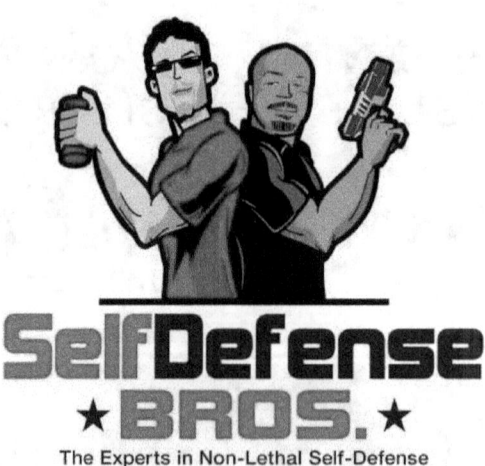

The Experts in Non-Lethal Self-Defense

For all of the people in the world who have suffered from crime or have been fortunate to have prevented or stopped it, this book is dedicated to you.

CONTENTS

INTRODUCTION 1

SECTION 1 Awareness of Self 3

Personal Safety Tip #1: An aware mind is key to safety. 3

Personal Safety Tip #2: Knowledge is power! 4

Personal Safety Tip #3: Have a warrior mindset. 4

Personal Safety Tip #4: Be careful of whom you trust. 5

SECTION 2 Avoiding the Crime 7

Personal Safety Tip #5: Dress consciously. 7

Personal Safety Tip #6: Watch the alcohol. 8

Personal Safety Tip #7: Use crime maps to see *good* and *bad* areas. 9

SECTION 3 Preventing the Crime 11

Personal Safety Tip #8: Don't make yourself a target. 11

Personal Safety Tip #9: Don't be complacent. 12

Personal Safety Tip #10: Change up your routine. 13

Personal Safety Tip #11: Make eye contact! 13

Personal Safety Tip #12: Implement *target hardening*. 15

i

SECTION 4 Preparing for the Crime...17

Personal Safety Tip #13: Always have an exit plan. 17

Personal Safety Tip #14: Don't rely on the police. 18

Personal Safety Tip #15: ALWAYS trust your gut feeling. 20

SECTION 5 Addressing the Crime 23

Personal Safety Tip #17: ALWAYS fight back or run!....................... 23

Personal Safety Tip #18: Never turn your back on someone. 25

Personal Safety Tip #19: Don't scream "Help!"............................... 25

Personal Safety Tip #20: Report the crime! 27

SECTION 6 Use of Force 29

Personal Safety Tip #21: Understand the *Use of Force Continuum*. 29

Personal Safety Tip #22: Don't rely on a gun for self-defense. 31

SECTION 7 Know the Laws 33

Personal Safety Tip #23: Be aware of your state's laws & regulations 33

Personal Safety Tip #24: Know your pepper sprays. 35

Personal Safety Tip #25: Know your electroshock weapons. 37

CONCLUSION...39

BIBLIOGRAPHY 41

RESOURCES 45

ABOUT THE AUTHOR 53

WARNING & DISCLAIMER

This book describes tips gathered based on the author's experiences as an instructor and consultant. The author is not a lawyer and any advice expressed therein should not be taken as such. If you require a lawyer's assessment regarding said information, please consult one.

Although every effort has been made to ensure the accuracy of the contents of this book, errors and omissions may occur. The publisher assumes no responsibility for any damages arising from the use of this book, or alleged to have resulted in connection with this book.

This book is not completely comprehensive; it merely offers general guidelines or tips with which to go by. Some readers of this book may wish to consult with additional books and advice before developing their personal safety plan. Additional personal safety sources are listed in the Resources portion at the end of this book.

INTRODUCTION

According to the Federal Bureau of Investigation (FBI), a violent crime occurred every 26.3 seconds and a property crime occurred every 3.9 seconds in 2015, within the United States.[1] That is a lot of crime! But how can we put all of this into perspective? Or better yet, how can we prevent or minimize the frequency of criminal activity?

You might be surprised to know that most crimes are not planned, but are actually *crimes of opportunity*. Many criminal acts, particularly burglary and robbery are all about taking advantage of vulnerable targets at a specific point in time. The bad thing about all these crimes is that we tend to put ourselves in vulnerable situations. The good news is that we can do something about it!

---

[1] 2015 Crime Clock Statistics (2015). Retrieved from:
https://ucr.fbi.gov/crime-in-the-u.s/2015/crime-in-the-u.s.-2015/resource-pages/crime-clock

This book was written to provide the most crucial tips for preserving one's personal safety. Some subjects of interest will sound familiar and make common sense while others will not. But you can be assured of one thing: **these tips can most certainly save your life!** The most important thing is to be aware and be prepared with the information you gather herein. At the end of this book there will be several resources you can utilize to further your crime prevention toolkit.

Overall, my goal here is to give you the tools and education you need to prevent crime and live a safer life. That is what I have dedicated myself to as a crime prevention practitioner and consultant. If the information I provide can save at least one life, then I have achieved my goal.

If you enjoy this book, please give it a rating on Amazon or in other venues. Every review, good or bad, helps me see what I can improve upon.

SECTION 1

Awareness of Self

The first important step to preserving one's personal safety is *awareness of self*. That involves knowing your inner self: mindfulness, knowledge, confidence and knowing whom to trust. Every piece is a critical part of your crime prevention toolkit. Let's go over four different personal safety tips that comprise this.

Personal Safety Tip #1
An aware mind is key to safety.

The greatest tool you can have is not pepper spray or a gun, but your MIND! A clear, focused mind that has a heightened sense of awareness is your BEST preventative measure against crime. That means being aware of your surroundings, honing your self-confidence and understanding that you can be affected by crime just as easily as the next person. Train your mind to be your first level of defense.

Best advice: **STAY AWARE AND BE PREPARED**

Personal Safety Tip #2
<u>Knowledge is power!</u>

Regardless of the tool you have, whether it is pepper spray or even a gun, make sure you KNOW how it works. A gun, for example, requires that you understand how to shoot, when to shoot, how to inspect it, how to react to a threat and to have constant practice firing it. Pepper spray and stun guns are no different. Be prepared! Learn how and what to carry, how to deploy, engage threats, be aware of expiration dates (pepper spray) and laws & regulations. Being prepared can save your life!

Personal Safety Tip #3
<u>Have a warrior mindset.</u>

Understand that when presented with a threat your goal is to **FIGHT** and to **WIN!** To properly survive in this world, one must develop a **WARRIOR MINDSET**. This applies not only to social or financial survival, but survival of the body and soul as well.

The most important thing to do is to hone your mind, to tell yourself that you are **NOT** a victim and will **NEVER** be one! Strengthen your mental awareness and master the tools (whether martial arts, self-defense products or a gun) you utilize to protect yourself from harm. When addressing a threat, do not cower in fear; make your enemy fear you instead: by being confident, laser-focused and proud.

Personal Safety Tip #4
Be careful of whom you trust.

Did you know that most crimes tend to be committed by people you know rather than complete strangers?[2] This is especially true for young people, aged 20-24. Sexual assault tends to be the most predominant, but non-stranger crime also includes other acts of violence as well.

Remember the common advice, "Don't talk to strangers"? It would be more appropriate to say, **"Be careful of your friends."** Frightening that those close to you are more likely to stab you in the back than some random criminal, right? Don't be paranoid; just keep this information in the back of your mind at all times. **Trust, but never trust fully.** Do not be so naïve to think that a relative or close friend would never act abnormally.

---

[2] Stranger vs. Non-Stranger Crime (2016, August 19). Retrieved from: https://threatanalysis.com/2016/08/19/stranger-v-non-stranger-crime

SECTION 2

Avoiding the Crime

The first thing that can be done in regards to crime is simply to try and avoid it when possible. That takes precautionary planning, but the sort that might ruin fun for some. Clothes, alcohol and knowing your geography all play a pivotal role in whether or not crime will strike. Be aware that the following tips will not guarantee you can avoid criminal activity; they will only help to minimize the chance of it.

Personal Safety Tip #5
Dress consciously.

Just as a predator in the wild seeks out prey that is the most vulnerable and easy to catch, so does a human predator think and act the same way. There is a lot of controversy behind the idea that women should not wear revealing clothing, so as to protect them from sexual assault...effectively shifting the blame from the criminal to the victim. But there are legitimate points to be made.

For one, wearing tight dresses and/or heels automatically makes you a target because you can't run away so easily. Dressing ostentatiously can attract unwanted attention from people (predators) who have bad intentions. It's really no different than being under the influence of alcohol; **again, easy target.**

Everyone should be able to wear what they want, but that does not change the harshness of reality and what actions others decide to take. Point is, take HEED and be cautious. If you decide to go all out, be prepared with a backup plan and defensive measures.

Personal Safety Tip #6
<u>Watch the alcohol.</u>

Alcohol is one of the greatest threats to one's personal safety, especially for young women in college. They tend to be the most vulnerable due to the college party environment and a tendency to have a relatively carefree lifestyle. Being inebriated inhibits judgment and the ability to see warning signs. It also significantly limits your ability to fight back.

Watch the alcohol; don't drink more than what you can handle, regardless of the social scene you're in. Limit yourself to no more than what will allow you to properly coordinate, balance and react to threats. **ALWAYS** watch your drinks and never let anyone make one for you, save for a bartender. Always have a very close friend that can keep an eye on you and have the tools and knowledge so as to be prepared for any subsequent threats after the bar scene is over.

Personal Safety Tip #7
Use crime maps to see *good* and *bad* areas.

When traveling or planning to go to a new area, whether in a new part of your city or out of state, always assess where you are heading to. There are a number of websites that provide public crime map data that you can utilize to see what issues are in your location. This will help you prepare for, or even avoid, certain parts of a city.

Public crime map data is especially helpful when looking for a new home. Real estate agents are forbidden by Fair Housing Law to disclose *how safe* an area is or what the demographics are. You will have to search that information out for yourself. City Data is another useful resource for learning which cities or neighborhoods are safer (no place is truly safe to live in).

The crime map system that I highly recommend is LexisNexus Community Crime Map (formerly RAIDS). If nothing pops up in your city, then your local police department does not have their data sourced with them and use another provider instead.

Look for other crime maps online or simply contact your police department to see which company they are working with for mapping their crime data.

SECTION 3

Preventing the Crime

Preventing crime is your main objective, especially when avoiding it usually proves to be difficult. Crime prevention works by eliminating threat vulnerabilities, whether in physical infrastructure or in behavioral patterns. That includes doing things that make you a harder target, not being complacent, changing up your routine, making eye contact with others and making your property more difficult to breach.

Personal Safety Tip #8
<u>Don't make yourself a target.</u>

Remember that most criminal acts are *crimes of opportunity*. For a criminal that means having the opportunity to exploit any vulnerability at a given time, whether that means robbing someone who has their face buried in their phone and headphones in their ears or taking advantage of an unlocked car or home with an open window. Simply put, these types of situations make you or your property an easy target. And criminals **ALWAYS** look for the most vulnerable targets.

Common sense goes a **LONG** way in preventing crime. If everyone did what they were supposed to, most street crime would drop. But the problem is that most of us get complacent. Being aware of your surroundings and keeping your property secure are all examples of good crime prevention.

Personal Safety Tip #9
Don't be complacent.

Complacency is literally the **BIGGEST** killer. Most of us operate through the mindset of, "Nothing (crime) will happen to me because I live or work in a safe area." That could mean college, an upper-middle class neighborhood, etc.

Complacency means lowering your **GUARD** because you are comfortable with your circumstances. But doing so makes you vulnerable, effectively placing a big **TARGET** on your back. Don't do it, because it can and will get you killed!

Remember that an ounce of **PREVENTION** is worth a pound of cure. And prevention requires lack of complacency. A wise man always told me, "Live life with as few regrets as possible." Do not allow your sense of complacency to be your biggest regret, because you may not even live to regret it.

Personal Safety Tip #10
<u>Change up your routine.</u>

Some people, stalkers especially, take advantage of people because they know their exact schedule. Assassins and other ill-intentioned persons work in the same fashion. While holding a consistent schedule, like going for a run around the lake every Tuesday night at 8pm, is convenient and keeps your life structured...it can also make you or your property an **EASY** target.

Routinization is a favorite part of life for the experienced criminal. Try to take different routes or alter your schedule slightly every week in order to keep the bad guys on their toes. This will make it more difficult for people who want to target you.

Personal Safety Tip #11
<u>Make eye contact!</u>

It is our natural instinct as humans to look away when we are approaching or passing by other people. We do this because we do not want to bring attention to ourselves or we are simply too embarrassed to make eye contact. But did you know that criminals can take advantage of this?

Let me tell you a story about my friend Bianca.

Bianca was waiting at a bus stop at a college. A man made multiple comments to her, telling her she was pretty and such. She said "Okay" and tried to ignore him, putting her head down and not making eye contact. The guy got irritated and eventually ended up walking off.

Now, **the next day Bianca saw on the news that the SAME guy and four other men sexually assaulted a college student.** She could have ended up the same way! But the worst part about the interaction?

She had her head down!

I have seen **SO many women put their heads down in passing when walking by me.** It's a reflex women have in order to avoid scrutiny or to avoid contact altogether...

BUT THIS CAN GET YOU KILLED!

Someone could easily rob you if he or she noticed that you weren't paying attention. Whether that means being occupied by your cell phone, headphones or just having your head down.

ALWAYS be aware of your surroundings! We humans have a natural tendency not to stare at people because it is considered rude or makes you come off as intimidating. I am the same way.

But you should PRACTICE scanning your area at all times. You don't have to stare, just take glances. Ignoring someone entirely might make you temporarily comfortable, but those blinders can get torn down in a bad way.

Looking away from a potential threat is to willingly blind yourself. It is no different than not listening to your *gut feeling*. Criminals can easily pickpocket/steal, grab you from behind, rob you, stalk you or even follow you home if you decide not to show some awareness. Simply looking someone in the eye in passing or turning your view to the rear tells people: **"I am AWARE and not an easy target; my eyes are on YOU!"** Awareness is the biggest threat to a criminal.

Personal Safety Tip #12
Implement *target hardening.*

If you are a homeowner, you should already know the basics on how to keep a good home. But do you know how to *harden* your property, to make it less vulnerable to crime by burglars and thieves? **Target hardening** is reflective of what is known as, in the field of crime prevention, Crime Prevention through Environmental Design (CPTED). It is the process of making a physical structure more secure and less prone to criminal activity.

Tips:

- Trim your bushes and refrain from using walls around your property; they make **PERFECT** hiding places for burglars.

- Install a home security system, either automated or DIY (do-it-yourself) and place a sign outside your home; burglars are less tempted to assault a home that could get them caught.

- Lock **ALL** doors and entryways: front & back doors, garage doors and windows. Burglars look for easy entry; don't give them the opportunity!

SECTION 4

Preparing for the Crime

Preparing for the crime is essential. If you are unable to avoid it or prevent it, you had better be prepared to address it. That means: always having a structured exit plan for escape, not relying on the police for your personal safety, always trusting your inner instincts or gut feeling and being aware of reaction time when engaging an assailant. An ounce of prevention may be worth a pound of cure, but an ounce of preparation is worth a pound of regret!

Personal Safety Tip #13
Always have an exit plan.

The most important part of being prepared is to have an **EXIT PLAN**. Martial arts schools and firearms trainers do not [typically] prepare you for real life situations. What if your attempts to subdue your attacker with hand-to-hand tactics fails? What if you freeze up with hesitation or miss your target with your gun? What are you going to do if things do not go as planned?! Not even pepper spray is foolproof!

The fact of the matter is that you need to have an escape plan ready in case things do not turn out as expected; because in life, many times they never do. As a good friend always says, "While they're playing checkers, I'm playing chess." It is **CRUCIAL** to always be one step ahead of your assailant! Because you can be sure that they have some backup plan, depending on their skill level.

Personal Safety Tip #14
<u>Don't rely on the police.</u>

Many of us, depending on our background, are raised from an early age to rely on the police. "The police protect us!" is the common thought process when crime is afoot. But there are **TWO** problems with this belief.

1. The average response time for 911 calls is 10 minutes![3] As they say, "When seconds count the police are only minutes away." 10 minutes is a **LONG** time to wait when you are being attacked.

---

[3] Pendleton, Kara. (2016, March). Here's How Long on Average It Takes for Police to Respond to a 911 Call. Retrieved from: http://self-defense-mind-body-spirit.com/average-police-response-time.html

2.   The police are **NOT** legally required to protect you, an "individual citizen", from crime.[4] If you wind up being sexually assaulted or even murdered, the police **CANNOT** be held liable for what transpired. This has been proven in over a decade of court cases.

For example, on February 12th, 2011 Maksim Gelman went on a stabbing spree in a New York City subway station. Joseph Lozito was stabbed seven times in his attempt to subdue Gelman, all while two NYPD police officers stood by and watched. Lozito later sued the NYPD and the City of New York for failing to intervene. City lawyer David Santoro stated that **"under well-established law, the police are not liable for such incidents."**[5] This statement validates the importance of self-reliance over government dependence.

I am not discounting the importance of calling 911 for help; just don't rely on it as your lifeline. We encourage everyone to be their OWN *first responder*, to fight back and not be a victim! Take a proactive approach rather than a reactive one through

---

[4] Faircloth, Ulrich. (2012, November 12). Don't Rely on the Police to Save You – Protect Yourself!. Retrieved from: http://srselfdefense.com/blog/no-duty-to-protect/

[5] Bonlello, Kathlanne. (2013, January 27). City says cops had no duty to protect subway hero who subdued killer. Retrieved from:
http://nypost.com/2013/01/27/city-says-cops-had-no-duty-to-protect-subway-hero-who-subdued-killer

the police. By the time they get to you, you may already have passed on. It is your responsibility to account for your own safety.

Personal Safety Tip #15
ALWAYS trust your gut feeling.

If something doesn't feel right, it usually isn't. Our bodies have a natural way of telling us when a situation just isn't good. Your instincts are a far better judge of character than what your mind or logic can provide in regards to a stranger.

Point is, **ALWAYS** trust your instincts or your gut feeling because it is far better to be safe than sorry. It is better to overreact and spray a suspected criminal with pepper spray and apologize later than hesitate and possibly lose your dignity or your life. Remember, "Better to be judged by 12 than carried by 6." A dead person cannot feel regret.

Personal Safety Tip #16
Be wary of reaction time.

Did you know that most assaults happen within 6-8 feet? Or that an assailant can close a distance of 21 feet in about 1.5 seconds?[6] Reaction time is a BIG deal in self-defense. The **reactionary gap** refers to the amount of time it takes for you to recognize, engage and neutralize a threat. It is the proper distance you must keep between yourself and the assailant in order to properly react and handle the threat successfully.

The #1 issue that I see with people who utilize pepper spray is, aside from holding and deploying it, how they carry it. I have seen SO many instances of women that keep their spray in their purse. This does you **NO GOOD!** Digging to the bottom of your purse to grab your pepper spray to fend off an attacker decreases your reactionary time substantially. An assailant is not going to just wait to let you get your defensive weapon out.

If you must have spray in your purse, have a clip or key chain spray that you can attach to an inside or outside pocket for easy access. Proper awareness and easy access to your pepper spray, stun gun or other personal safety device is crucial in any self-defense situation.

---

[6] Borelli, Frank. (2001, July). Twenty-one Feet is Way Too Close. Retrieved from:
https://www.ncjrs.gov/App/Publications/abstract.aspx?ID=203269

SECTION 5

Addressing the Crime

Now this is why preparing is so important. Eventually at some point in life you will wind up in a situation where you are caught in the midst of a crime and will have to address it or engage an assailant. Handling the crime involves fighting back or running, not turning your back on someone, not screaming for help and making sure to report the crime immediately after the altercation. These tips will help you get out of a situation better than doing the opposite of what is proposed.

Personal Safety Tip #17
<u>ALWAYS fight back or run!</u>

When faced with a threat, you have choices to make. Do you plead with your attacker, give in to their demands or resist with force? Believe it or not, in most situations you should **FIGHT BACK or try to RUN!**

"Never underestimate the power of running"[7], especially when encountering a threat with a firearm. You have a much higher chance of survival trying to run from an assailant versus going with them in a car and quite possibly disappearing forever. Under stressful conditions your average criminal is going to have poor accuracy. Even police officers have difficulty hitting their targets at times. Fact is, better to get grazed than leave your life in the hands of your attacker. Just try not to run in a straight line.

Fighting back is the other option. But this should be done with your best judgment, considering the circumstances. If your assailant wants your wallet or other valuables, just give them up; your life is worth far more. If someone is trying to sexually assault you on the other hand, best to **FIGHT BACK!** The more difficult you can make things for your assailant, the better chance you have of coming out alive as well as being mentally and physically sound.

---

[7] Lashway, Zachery. (2016, September 7). Tips for Kids on Staying Safe from Predators. Retrieved from: http://www.kare11.com/news/tips-for-kids-on-staying-safe-from-predators/315323544

Personal Safety Tip #18
<u>Never turn your back on someone.</u>

Ever heard of the term "watch your six"? In the military that means watch your back. This is crucial for the everyday person, especially. Your blind spot, the rear, is your most vulnerable area. **ALWAYS** pay attention to people who are following you. Periodically turn your head to check and see; especially if things just don't feel right (your gut feeling).

One very important thing to keep in mind during an altercation: if you manage to get your attacker down and you think that they are immobilized, **DO NOT TURN YOUR BACK** when trying to get away. Walk backwards or side-ways so that you can keep an eye on the assailant. If you plan on turning your back regardless, do not do so until you have a safe distance of about 25 feet away from the attacker. You might think he or she is down and out, but that could very well change once you turn around.

Personal Safety Tip #19
<u>Don't scream "Help!"</u>

During an attack, it is a common response to reach out to others for help; typically, by screaming *help!* But the word **help** is just as effective as a car alarm screeching: people will unconsciously phase it out. Yelling "fire" or "there's a bomb!" will at least get people's attention and have them react quickly.

The other important thing to remember is that even if you reach out for help, you may not receive it. In 1964 Kitty Genovese was stabbed to death outside of her apartment in New York City, despite her call for help and the number of witnesses that saw the crime in progress.

The **Genovese Effect** or **Bystander Effect** is a social phenomenon that refers to situations in which help is not offered to someone in need of it, from people nearby. It is typically explained by *diffusion of responsibility,* which means that help is less likely to be offered, based on the number of people present, because there is an expectation that someone else will assist instead.[8]

Ultimately **human beings are more concerned about not getting involved in an incident rather than helping another person.** These days a person is likely to whip out their phone and record quicker than offering help This is why you cannot solely rely on the police **OR** other everyday people, because you could wind up dead or seriously injured.

---

[8] Cherry, Kendra (2016, June 22). What is Diffusion of Responsibility? Retrieved from: https://www.verywell.com/what-is-diffusion-of-responsibility-2795095

Personal Safety Tip #20
Report the crime!

Did you know that most sexual assaults go unreported? That's about 66% or 2 out of 3 according to RAINN.[9] Most people do not want to report a violent crime due to fear, shame or trauma. Much of it also comes down to lack of details on the assailant. Reporting a crime **IMMEDIATELY** after the attack has occurred and with as much detail is the best course of action.

A criminal act, whether someone did a hit & run with their vehicle or if you were robbed, tends to happen so fast that we tend to forgo the details of the situation. We are more concerned with the present circumstances rather than what should be done in the aftermath.

After a crime has occurred, contact the police **IMMEDIATELY**. Be prepared to give as many details as possible: time & location of the incident, physical description of the assailant, an explanation of what happened, eye witness testimony (if applicable), etc. **Never wait to file a report**, as information is fresher on the mind right after the event.

---

[9] Rape, Abuse & Incest National Network. (Unknown). The Criminal Justice System: Statistics. Retrieved from: https://www.rainn.org/statistics/criminal-justice-system

SECTION 6

Use of Force

When engaging a threat one must be aware of the level of force that can be used. Believe it or not, but we as regular civilians have to follow a use of force policy similar to that of police officers. The only differences are that we do not have a union to protect us and the force we use is to escape a violent encounter rather than to subdue a criminal. That is what it is crucial to understand the concept of the *use of force continuum* and to know how problematic a gun is for use in self-defense.

Personal Safety Tip #21

Understand the *Use of Force Continuum.*

When picking a self-defense tool, whether it is a non-lethal or less-lethal choice such as pepper spray or a TASER or a lethal product like a gun or a knife, you should be aware of how the level of force applies in different circumstances. The **use of force continuum** applies to both law enforcement and civilians.

But unlike cops, everyday people like you and I do not have a union to protect us.

This is why understanding the use of force continuum is paramount to your overall safety, both in the street and in the courtroom. You cannot use excessive force against someone…even if they are attacking you.[10] That means, for example, using a firearm against an unarmed criminal. You can go overboard, but expect to explain, in court, the reasoning behind the level of force that you committed to.

The only exception is under special or ***exigent circumstances***. These could be if you were dealing with multiple assailants (e.g. "knock-out game" situation), your attacker was physically stronger than you or you feared for your life (e.g. George Zimmerman; poor case, but vindicated in a court of law). Even if you avoid being criminally charged, an assailant or their relatives could sue you in civil court for damages. This even occurred with a criminal who died while attempting to burglarize a fumigated home! His family tried to sue.

---

[10] Just be aware that I am **not** a lawyer; I say this only to make people aware of the liability involved.

Personal Safety Tip #22
<u>Don't rely on a gun for self-defense.</u>

When you say the word *self-defense,* most people think of martial arts (hand-to-hand) or a gun (weapon). Believe it or not (sorry, gun enthusiasts), a firearm is a very poor choice for your personal safety.[11] More than 91% of violent encounters will not involve a gun[12], so you are far better off using a non-lethal/less-lethal device like pepper spray for your personal safety. Not only that, but there are numerous problems involved with using a firearm. Your average person is not equipped to handle all of them.

Non-lethal or less-lethal self-defense is ideal for most situations. The fact is that 80% of the time you will be facing an unarmed assailant. If you are inclined to have a firearm for your protection, have it only as a back-up for when things require an upgrade to lethal force in order to neutralize the threat. Otherwise, stick with some variation of pepper spray.

---

[11] Faircloth, Ulrich (2012, November 17). Why Guns are a Poor Choice for Self-Defense. Retrieved from:
http://www.srselfdefense.com/blog/why-guns-are-a-poor-choice-for-selfdefense

[12] King, Russell (2016, June 30). The long-term solution to gun and other violence: Redefine manhood. Retrieved from:
http://host.madison.com/ct/opinion/column/russell-king-the-long-term-solution-to-gun-and-other/article_e82a95ae-ed21-5684-80a9-074bd0df47d3.html

SECTION 7

Know the Laws

Since I advocate the use of less-lethal weapons through Stun & Run Self Defense, I highly advise knowing your local, county and state laws regarding the usage of these devices. Laws on pepper spray and electroshock weapons (stun guns and TASERs) are the most common. Most people will buy one of these tools and not realize how restrictive their state laws might be regarding their use. This is why it is crucial to know the laws!

Personal Safety Tip #23
<u>Be aware of your state's laws & regulations.</u>

Folks here in Minnesota always ask, "Are stun guns legal?" or "Are pepper sprays legal?" And thankfully the answer is, "Yes and with no restrictions, unless you are a felon." Every state has different laws pertaining to self-defense products such as pepper spray, stun guns, TASERs, expandable batons and so on. Be aware of your state's restrictions!

Here are some of the WORST states (in my opinion) for less-lethal self-defense.

NEW YORK – Stun guns and TASERs are ILLEGAL in New York. Pepper sprays CANNOT be purchased online or by mail order. They can only be purchased from an in-state authorized pharmacist or firearms dealer. Expandable batons are ILLEGAL.

MASSACHUSETTS – Stun guns and TASERs are ILLEGAL in Massachusetts. Pepper sprays were once considered to be *ammunition* and an FOID card was required for purchase. Pepper spray CANNOT be purchased online or by mail order, only through an in-state authorized firearms dealer or pharmacist. Expandable batons are ILLEGAL.

NEW JERSEY – Stun guns and TASERs are ILLEGAL in New Jersey. Pepper spray is restricted to ¾ oz. Expandable batons are ILLEGAL.

HAWAII – Stun guns and TASERs are ILLEGAL in Hawaii. Pepper spray cannot be shipped from the Continental U.S.; must be purchased in-state due to federal regulations. Usage is restricted to ½ oz. Expandable batons are ILLEGAL.

WISCONSIN – This state has by far the most restrictions on pepper spray. Your pepper spray cannot contain tear gas (CS/CN), cannot be camouflaged (e.g. no pepper spray bracelets), must have a safety feature to prevent accidental discharge, must be no more than 10% OC formulation, no more than 2 oz in weight and MUST have a minimum effective range of 6 feet but no more than 20 feet (e.g. no large bear spray canisters). Stun guns and TASERs require an FOID card. Expandable batons: *possibly* legal or illegal depending on state statute.

Personal Safety Tip #24
Know your pepper sprays.

I always tell people that there is a **LOT** to pepper spray besides just buying a unit and using it against an attacker. One of the biggest things is being aware of **what type of spray pattern or dispersal pattern** you should have in a defense spray. It all depends on your overall circumstances or what you expect to need. There are four different types: stream, fog, foam and gel.

Stream – The most common spray pattern, in use by police and civilians. Comes out straight like a water gun. **User must have good aim and go for the eyes.** There is less blowback or cross-contamination with this spray in windy situations or indoor areas compared to other dispersal types.

Fog – Similar to a cone mist, fogger pepper sprays come out like a thick fog. **They are excellent when facing multiple assailants.** There is no need to aim; just spray in the direction of the assailant(s) to create a barrier. The droplets in the spray are much finer and as a result, fog types are easily breathed in. They are highly susceptible to blowback and cross-contamination, however.

Foam – Sprays with this dispersal pattern eject like a fire extinguisher, covering an attacker with foam that irritates the skin. No fumes are emitted, unlike a stream or fog, which makes **the foam pattern great for enclosed areas like hospitals or schools.** The disadvantage is that it can be wiped off by the attacker and thrown back at you.

Gel – This is our go-to dispersal pattern for dealing with single targets. A gel is sprayed, which sticks like glue to the target. **If the assailant tries to get it off it digs deeper into the skin, causing greater pain.** No fumes, so no worries about cross-contamination or blowback. Like the stream, the face must be targeted for maximum effect.

Personal Safety Tip #25

Know your electroshock weapons.

Like pepper spray and *Mace*, you should also know that there are clear distinctions between two of the most commonly known electroshock weapons: stun guns and TASERs, the most popular brand of electronic control device (ECD).

Stun Guns – Despite the name, stun guns do not actually look like a gun. **They are close-contact devices that emit a high voltage, low amperage shock to cause pain and disorient an attacker.** Unlike the TASER, the stun gun relies on pain compliance to work and is often ineffective against persons who have a high pain tolerance. This is particularly true for people under the influence of drugs or alcohol. It must be held directly on the skin for 3-5 seconds in order to be effective. They come in various forms: cell phones, walking canes, flashlights, lipstick, etc.

TASER – The Tom A. Swift Electric Rifle (TASER) looks more like a gun. It shoots barbed prongs in the shape of fish hooks, ejected by nitrogen, up to 35 feet away (15 foot maximum for civilians). **When both prongs hit the target they involuntarily lock the muscles up in the human body by way of *neuro-muscular incapacitation (NMI).*** This effect only works if both prongs hit the body. The TASER's *drive stun* capability turns it into a stun gun at close range.

CONCLUSION

You can either try to avoid crime or prevent it. And the only way to do the latter is to prepare for it. If you get into a situation where you have an altercation with someone then do what you can to protect yourself and report it immediately after! Knowing how to defend yourself, whether through weapons or martial arts, is essential. You should know the laws of your state and apply them as needed, both in terms of use of force as well as self-defense tools.

In summary, the 25 personal safety tips we covered will help keep you safe from crime. The most critical element of all is awareness. If you are not aware of your surroundings, believe that you cannot be a target for criminal activity or lack self-awareness then you have failed to adequately prepare yourself for the dangers of our world. It is a scary place out there, but it does not have to be.

If you ever find yourself in a pinch, do not hesitate to utilize the Resources page of this book for help. Otherwise if you need some personal guidance, I am only a phone call away at 612-217-2335. I can help you with your issue at no charge if you mention having read this self-defense guide. If you are looking for personal safety courses, please check out our course offerings at www.stunrunacademy.com

Besides that, thank you for purchasing this book. I hope that it has helped you to be more aware of your surroundings and to stay safe!

BIBLIOGRAPHY

1. 2015 Crime Clock Statistics (2015). Retrieved from: https://ucr.fbi.gov/crime-in-the-u.s/2015/crime-in-the-u.s.-2015/resource-pages/crime-clock.

2. Stranger vs. Non-Stranger Crime (2016, August 19). Retrieved from: https://www.threatanalysis.com/2016/08/19/stranger-v-non-stranger-crime

3. Pendleton, Kara. (2016, March). Here's How Long on Average It Takes for Police to Respond to a 911 Call. Retrieved from: http://www.self-defense-mind-body-spirit.com/average-police-response-time.html

4. Faircloth, Ulrich. (2012, November 12). Don't Rely on the Police to Save You – Protect Yourself!. Retrieved from: http://www.srselfdefense.com/blog/no-duty-to-protect/

5. Bonlello, Kathlanne. (2013, January 27). City says cops had no duty to protect subway hero who subdued killer. Retrieved from: http://nypost.com/2013/01/27/city-says-cops-had-no-duty-to-protect-subway-hero-who-subdued-killer/

6. Borelli, Frank. (2001, July). Twenty-one Feet is Way Too Close. Retrieved from: https://www.ncjrs.gov/App/Publications/abstract.aspx?ID=203269

7. Lashway, Zachery. (2016, September 7). Tips for Kids on Staying Safe from Predators. Retrieved from: http://www.kare11.com/news/tips-for-kids-on-staying-safe-from-predators/315323544

8. Cherry, Kendra (2016, June 22). What is Diffusion of Responsibility? Retrieved from: https://www.verywell.com/what-is-diffusion-of-responsibility-2795095

9. Rape, Abuse & Incest National Network. (Unknown). The Criminal Justice System: Statistics. Retrieved from: https://www.rainn.org/statistics/criminal-justice-system

10. Just be aware that I am **not** a lawyer; I say this only to make people aware of the liability involved.

11. Faircloth, Ulrich (2012, November 17). Why Guns are a Poor Choice for Self-Defense. Retrieved from: http://www.srselfdefense.com/blog/why-guns-are-a-poor-choice-for-selfdefense/

12. King, Russell (2016, June 30). The long-term solution to gun and other violence: Redefine manhood. Retrieved from: http://host.madison.com/ct/opinion/column/russell-king-the-long-term-solution-to-gun-and-other/article_e82a95ae-ed21-5684-80a9-074bd0df47d3.html

RESOURCES

<u>Domestic Abuse & Sexual Assault</u>

National Coalition Against Domestic Violence (NCADV)

NCADV's Main Office

One Broadway, Suite B210

Denver, CO 80203

303-839-1852

mainoffice@ncadv.org

www.ncadv.org

The National Coalition Against Domestic Violence (NCADV) has been working to help and protect men and women from domestic abuse since 1978. They actively work to influence public policy in this area, as well as to provide programs and education for those in need. NCADV offers a ton of resources and support.

Rape, Abuse & Incest National Network (RAINN)

Rape, Abuse & Incest National Network

1220 L St NW #505

Washington, DC 20005

202-544-1034

www.rainn.org

RAINN (Rape, Abuse & Incest National Network) is the nation's largest anti-sexual violence organization in the United States. It has helped more than 2.4 million people since 1994. They specialize in crisis intervention and operate the National Sexual Assault helpline for those in need of assistance, in conjunction with more than 1,000 local sexual assault providers across the country to provide services.

Personal Safety

Project for Pride in Living (PPL)

Project for Pride in Living

1035 East Franklin Avenue

Minneapolis, MN 55404

612-445-5100

www.ppl-inc.org

Project for Pride in Living (PPL) is an excellent resource for anyone looking for help with employment or housing, but also personal safety. They have a list of personal safety resources on their website. You can utilize their Personalized Safety Plan as a guideline for what to look out for.

Arming Women Against Rape & Endangerment (AWARE)

We are AWARE
PO Box 245
Ashland, MA 01721

info@aware.org
www.aware.org

Arming Women Against Rape & Endangerment (AWARE) is a non-profit that provides great material for women who are in need of personal safety advice. They go over the importance of self-defense, tools that can be utilized and offer an abundance of information on how to tackle violent encounters.

Stun & Run Academy

support@stunrunacademy.com
www.stunrunacademy.com

Stun & Run Academy is our resource for online courses. We currently offer the following classes, but more are being created:

- Introduction to Non-Lethal Self-Defense
- Pepper Spray 101: How to Protect Yourself at a Distance
- Electroshock Weapons: Stun Guns & TASERs

The material covered in these courses is unique; there are no other online courses like them. **Mention this book when emailing to get a special discount code.** Be on the lookout for books and audiobooks on these topics as well!

If for some reason the website is not up, you can find these courses on Udemy.com:

https://www.udemy.com/user/ulrich-faircloth-2/

Community Crime Maps

LexisNexus Community Crime Map

www.communitycrimemap.com

Crime Reports

www.crimereports.com

Crime Mapping

www.crimemapping.com

Crime maps are an excellent way of compiling and representing crime that has occurred over a period of time. I highly recommend using them if you are planning on purchasing a home and are unsure of how the neighborhood is or if you are going to a new area for whatever reason. Just be aware that this is merely spatial data based on what has been reported.

Self-Defense Products

Stun & Run Self Defense LLC

2122 Grand Ave S.
APT 305
Minneapolis, MN 55405

612-217-2335
www.stunrun.com

If you are looking for self-defense tools such as pepper spray, stun guns and TASER devices then Stun & Run Self Defense is your one-stop shop. We also carry survival gear, spy gear and tactical equipment for security guards, police and bounty hunters. Sign up for the email list to get access to tons of great crime prevention information, especially in regards to less-lethal self-defense options.

<u>Crime Prevention Consulting</u>

Self Defense Bros.

2122 Grand Ave S.
APT 305
Minneapolis, MN 55405

612-217-2146
www.selfdefensebros.com

If you are looking for personal safety training for your personnel, clientele or require a detailed security assessment of your property then the Self Defense Bros. are your best bet. We provide crime prevention consulting for for-profit companies, nonprofit organizations and home owners located in the Twin Cities. We are willing to travel to other parts of Minnesota, as well as to nearby states such as Wisconsin and North Dakota to provide training.

Crime Doctor

213-537-3505

www.crimedoctor.com

Chris McGoey is a crime prevention expert and security consultant who has over 46 years of education and experience, in addition to thousands of hours in specialized training. He is a go-to person for personal safety advice, security consulting and circumstances requiring a security expert witness. Mr. McGoey provides a wealth of information in the security field.

ABOUT THE AUTHOR

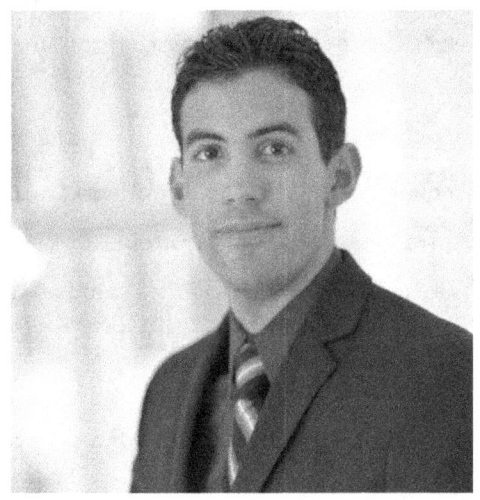

Ulrich Faircloth is a crime prevention practitioner and consultant. His passion for crime prevention began while working as a crime prevention intern for the Minneapolis Police Department. He later served as a non-sworn community service officer (CSO) with the department for a short period, but ultimately decided that he wanted to be more involved on a community level. This decision led him to focus on proactive solutions to addressing crime.

Ulrich is the founder and co-owner of Stun & Run Self Defense LLC, an ecommerce store intent on "preventing crime and saving lives" by giving people the tools and education they need to protect themselves and their loved ones. He is also the cofounder of Self Defense Bros., a crime prevention consultancy that specializes in less-lethal self-defense and personal safety training for local businesses, non-profit organizations and universities.

Ulrich received a B.A. in Sociology from Beloit College in 2012. He is a certified OC (oleoresin capsicum) Aerosol Instructor through TJA Use of Force Training, Inc. and has five years of experience in the private security field. He is actively working on his crime prevention specialist certifications. He is originally from Lumberton, NC but now resides in Minneapolis, MN.

Learn more about Ulrich at:

www.stunrun.com

www.selfdefensebros.com